SAXENDA USAGE MEDICAL GUIDE

A Step-By-Step Manual For Optimal Usage And Dosage With Utilization Strategies For Enhanced Effectiveness And Safety

CONTENTS

I. Introduction

II. Understanding Saxenda

III. Usage Guidelines

IV. Dosage Guidelines

V. How to Use Saxenda for Optimal Results

VI. Ensuring Effectiveness and Safety

VII. Conclusion

INTRODUCTION

Welcome to "Saxenda Usage Med Guide," your comprehensive companion to navigating the world of Saxenda – a groundbreaking pharmaceutical treatment designed to assist individuals in their weight loss journey. In this guide, we embark on a journey through the intricacies of Saxenda, shedding light on its mechanism, importance, and practical application.

A. Brief Overview of Saxenda:

Saxenda, a brand name for liraglutide, stands as a beacon of hope for those striving to achieve sustainable weight loss. As a glucagon-like peptide-1 (GLP-1) receptor agonist, Saxenda operates by mimicking the actions of natural hormones in the body, particularly those that regulate appetite and metabolism. By enhancing feelings of fullness and reducing hunger, Saxenda aids individuals in managing their weight effectively.

B. Importance of Understanding Usage and Dosage Guidelines:

Navigating the landscape of pharmaceutical interventions necessitates a profound understanding of usage and dosage guidelines. In the case of Saxenda, adherence to prescribed dosages and administration protocols is paramount for ensuring optimal results and minimizing potential risks. Through a comprehensive grasp of usage guidelines, individuals can harness the full potential of Saxenda while mitigating the likelihood of adverse effects.

C. Purpose of the Medical Guide:

The "Saxenda Usage Med Guide" serves as an indispensable resource, equipping readers with the knowledge and insights needed to embark on their Saxenda journey with confidence and clarity. From elucidating the intricacies of Saxenda's mechanism of action to providing practical tips for incorporating it into daily life, this guide is tailored to empower individuals with the information they need to make informed decisions regarding their health and well-being.

Join us as we delve into the realms of Saxenda, unlocking its transformative potential and paving the way toward a healthier, happier future. Let this guide be your compass on the path to weight management success.

UNDERSTANDING SAXENDA

A. Brief Overview of Saxenda:

Saxenda, a brand name for liraglutide, is an FDA-approved medication primarily used for weight management in adults with obesity or those who are overweight with at least one weight-related comorbidity. It belongs to a class of medications called glucagon-like peptide-1 (GLP-1) receptor agonists, which work by mimicking the effects of a naturally occurring hormone in the body called GLP-1.

Unlike many weight-loss medications, Saxenda is not an appetite suppressant. Instead, it works by slowing down the emptying of the stomach, making you feel fuller for longer periods. Additionally, Saxenda may also help regulate blood sugar levels, which can be beneficial for individuals with type 2 diabetes.

B. Importance of Understanding Usage and Dosage Guidelines:

Understanding the proper usage and dosage guidelines for Saxenda is crucial for achieving the desired results while minimizing the risk of adverse effects. Unlike over-the-counter supplements or medications, Saxenda is a prescription medication that should be used under the guidance of a healthcare professional.

The dosage of Saxenda is gradually increased over several weeks to minimize gastrointestinal side effects, such as nausea and diarrhea, which are common during the initial stages of treatment. Additionally, understanding how to properly administer Saxenda, either through the prefilled pen device or syringe, is essential for ensuring accurate dosing.

Furthermore, adherence to lifestyle modifications, such as a healthy diet and regular physical activity, is essential for maximizing the effectiveness of Saxenda. While Saxenda can aid in weight loss, it is not a standalone solution and should be used as part of a comprehensive weight management plan.

C. Purpose of the Medical Guide:

The medical guide accompanying Saxenda serves as a comprehensive resource for patients and healthcare providers alike. It provides detailed information on the medication's mechanism of action, dosage and administration guidelines, potential side effects, and tips for managing them.

Additionally, the medical guide outlines important safety information, contraindications, and precautions for use, helping both patients and healthcare providers make informed decisions about Saxenda therapy. It also emphasizes the importance of regular follow-up appointments with a healthcare provider to monitor progress and adjust treatment as needed.

Overall, the medical guide serves as a valuable tool in ensuring the safe and effective use of Saxenda, empowering individuals to take control of their weight management journey while minimizing potential risks.

USAGE GUIDELINES

In the realm of pharmacotherapy, adherence to proper usage guidelines is paramount to ensure both efficacy and safety. Saxenda, a medication designed to aid in weight management, is no exception. Understanding who should utilize Saxenda, along with precautions, contraindications, and potential interactions, is essential for both healthcare providers and patients alike.

A. Who Should Use Saxenda?

Saxenda is indicated for individuals struggling with obesity or overweight, particularly those with a body mass index (BMI) of 30 kg/m² or higher, or with a BMI of 27 kg/m² or higher in the presence of at least one weight-related comorbidity, such as hypertension, type 2 diabetes, or dyslipidemia. It is intended for adults aged 18 and older.

B. Precautions and Contraindications:

While Saxenda can be a valuable tool in weight management, it is not without risks. Certain precautions and contraindications must be carefully considered before initiating therapy. Patients with a history of pancreatitis should avoid Saxenda, as it has been associated with an increased risk of this condition. Additionally, individuals with a personal or family history of medullary thyroid carcinoma (MTC) or multiple endocrine neoplasia syndrome type 2 (MEN 2) should not use Saxenda due to its potential to stimulate thyroid C-cell tumors. Other contraindications include pregnancy, lactation, and known hypersensitivity to liraglutide or any of the product components.

C. Importance of Consulting a Healthcare Provider Before Use:

Prior to starting Saxenda, it is crucial for individuals to consult with a healthcare provider, preferably a physician experienced in obesity management. A thorough medical evaluation should be conducted to assess the patient's suitability for Saxenda therapy, taking into account their medical history, current medications, and any potential contraindications. This consultation also provides an opportunity for healthcare providers to educate patients about the benefits, risks, and expectations associated with Saxenda use.

D. Dosage Adjustments for Special Populations:

Special populations, such as the elderly and pediatric patients, may require dosage adjustments when using Saxenda. Elderly individuals, due to age-related changes in metabolism and renal function, may be more susceptible to adverse effects and may require lower initial doses, with gradual titration as tolerated. Pediatric patients have not been extensively studied with Saxenda and its safety and efficacy in this population have not been established; therefore, its use is not recommended in individuals under the age of 18.

E. Potential Drug Interactions to Be Aware Of:

As with any medication, Saxenda has the potential to interact with other drugs, potentially altering their efficacy or increasing the risk of adverse effects. Patients should inform their healthcare provider about all prescription, over-the-counter, and herbal medications they are taking, particularly other antidiabetic agents or medications affecting gastrointestinal motility, as these may interact with Saxenda. Close monitoring and dosage adjustments may be necessary when Saxenda is co-administered with such drugs.

In conclusion, adherence to Saxenda's usage guidelines is

essential to optimize its therapeutic benefits while minimizing risks. By carefully considering patient suitability, precautions, contraindications, and potential interactions, healthcare providers can facilitate safe and effective Saxenda therapy for individuals struggling with obesity or overweight.

DOSAGE GUIDELINES

In the journey towards weight management with Saxenda, understanding the dosage guidelines is crucial. This chapter delves into the recommended starting dose, titration schedule for dose escalation, maximum daily dose, administration instructions, and missed dose recommendations to ensure optimal utilization of this medical tool in your weight loss journey.

A. Recommended Starting Dose:

Embarking on the Saxenda regimen begins with careful consideration of the starting dose. For most individuals, the recommended starting dose is 0.6 mg once daily. This initial dose allows your body to acclimate to the medication gradually, minimizing the likelihood of adverse effects while still initiating the process of weight loss.

B. Titration Schedule for Dose Escalation:

As your body adjusts to Saxenda, gradual dose escalation is often necessary to achieve optimal results. After starting with the initial dose of 0.6 mg, the titration schedule involves increasing the dose in increments over time. Typically, the dose is increased by 0.6 mg weekly until the maintenance dose is reached.

C. Maximum Daily Dose:

Understanding the limits of Saxenda dosage is essential to ensure safety and efficacy. The maximum daily dose of Saxenda is 3 mg. Once the maintenance dose is achieved, it is imperative not to exceed this maximum limit to avoid potential adverse effects and maintain the intended therapeutic benefits.

D. Administration Instructions:

Administering Saxenda correctly is fundamental for its effectiveness. Saxenda comes in a pre-filled, multi-dose pen that delivers the medication subcutaneously (under the skin). To administer, follow these steps:

1. Select an injection site on your abdomen, thigh, or upper arm.

2. Clean the injection site with an alcohol swab and allow it to dry.

3. Hold the pen like a dart at a 90-degree angle to the skin.

4. Press the injection button firmly until the dose counter shows 0.

5. Continue to hold the button and count slowly to 5 to ensure the full dose is delivered.

6. Remove the needle from the skin and dispose of the pen properly.

Following these administration instructions ensures accurate dosing and consistent delivery of Saxenda.

E. Missed Dose Recommendations:

In the event of a missed dose, it is essential to take the next dose as soon as remembered, unless it is within 3 hours of the next scheduled dose. If this is the case, skip the missed dose and resume the regular dosing schedule. It is not advisable to double the dose to make up for a missed one, as this can increase the risk of side effects without providing additional benefits.

HOW TO USE SAXENDA FOR OPTIMAL RESULTS

Incorporating Saxenda into a weight loss regimen:

Successfully incorporating Saxenda into your weight loss regimen requires a comprehensive approach. This medication is not a standalone solution but rather a tool to support your efforts in achieving a healthier weight. It's essential to combine its use with lifestyle changes such as adopting a balanced diet and incorporating regular physical activity into your routine.

When starting Saxenda, it's crucial to set realistic weight loss goals and develop a plan that suits your individual needs. Consult with your healthcare provider to determine the appropriate dosage and schedule for taking Saxenda. Remember that consistency is key; adhere to your prescribed regimen to maximize the effectiveness of the medication.

Dietary and lifestyle recommendations:

Alongside Saxenda usage, making healthy dietary choices and adopting a more active lifestyle can significantly enhance your weight loss journey. Focus on consuming a well-rounded diet rich in fruits, vegetables, lean proteins, and whole grains while limiting processed foods and sugary beverages.

Incorporate regular physical activity into your routine, aiming for at least 30 minutes of moderate-intensity exercise most days of the week. This can include activities such as brisk walking, cycling, swimming, or strength training. Find activities that you enjoy and that fit into your schedule to increase adherence.

Monitoring progress and adjusting dosage as needed:

Regular monitoring of your progress is essential to assess the effectiveness of Saxenda and make any necessary adjustments. Keep track of your weight, dietary habits, physical activity, and any side effects you may experience. This information will help you and your healthcare provider evaluate your response to the medication and determine if any changes are needed.

Your healthcare provider may adjust your Saxenda dosage based on your weight loss progress and tolerance to the medication. It's important to follow their guidance closely and communicate any concerns or challenges you encounter along the way.

Addressing common challenges and side effects:

While Saxenda can be effective for weight loss, it may also present certain challenges and side effects. Common side effects include nausea, vomiting, diarrhea, and constipation. These symptoms usually improve over time as your body adjusts to the medication. However, if they persist or become severe, notify your healthcare provider.

To minimize side effects and maximize the effectiveness of Saxenda, it's essential to follow the prescribed dosage and administration instructions carefully. Additionally, staying hydrated, eating small, frequent meals, and avoiding high-fat foods can help alleviate gastrointestinal symptoms.

In conclusion, incorporating Saxenda into your weight loss regimen requires a multifaceted approach that includes dietary modifications, increased physical activity, regular monitoring, and open communication with your healthcare provider. By following these guidelines and addressing any challenges or side effects that arise, you can optimize your results and work towards achieving your weight loss goals with Saxenda.

ENSURING EFFECTIVENESS AND SAFETY

As you embark on your journey with Saxenda, it's crucial to understand the dynamics of its effectiveness and ensure your safety throughout the treatment process. This chapter will delve into the expected timeline for seeing results, signs of effectiveness, monitoring for adverse reactions, and the importance of reporting concerns to your healthcare provider.

A. Expected Timeline for Seeing Results:

Patience is key when starting Saxenda. While some individuals may notice changes sooner, it's essential to understand that weight loss doesn't happen overnight. Typically, noticeable weight loss can be observed within the first few weeks to months of starting Saxenda. However, individual responses may vary.

The timeline for seeing results largely depends on various factors, including your adherence to the prescribed regimen, lifestyle changes, and your body's unique response to the medication. Consistency in taking Saxenda as directed by your healthcare provider, combined with a balanced diet and regular physical activity, can enhance its effectiveness and expedite weight loss.

B. Signs of Effectiveness and When to Reassess Treatment:

Recognizing the signs of Saxenda's effectiveness is crucial for tracking your progress and determining if adjustments to your treatment plan are necessary. Some indicators of effectiveness may include:

Gradual Weight Loss: As you continue your Saxenda regimen, you may notice a steady decline in your weight over time.

Decreased Appetite: Many individuals experience a reduction in hunger and cravings, which can contribute to controlled eating habits.

Improved Metabolic Parameters: Alongside weight loss, improvements in metabolic markers such as blood sugar levels and cholesterol may indicate Saxenda's efficacy.

It's important to regularly reassess your treatment with your healthcare provider, typically every 16 weeks, to evaluate your progress and adjust your plan accordingly. During these follow-up appointments, your healthcare provider may consider factors such as weight loss trends, adherence to medication and lifestyle changes, and any potential side effects.

C. Monitoring for Adverse Reactions:

While Saxenda can be effective for weight loss, it's essential to be vigilant about potential adverse reactions that may arise during treatment. Common adverse reactions may include nausea, vomiting, diarrhea, constipation, abdominal pain, and low blood sugar levels (hypoglycemia).

Monitoring for adverse reactions involves paying close attention to how your body responds to Saxenda. If you experience any unusual or concerning symptoms, it's crucial to promptly report them to your healthcare provider. Additionally, monitoring your blood sugar levels regularly, especially if you have diabetes or are at risk of hypoglycemia, can help mitigate potential risks.

D. Reporting Concerns to Healthcare Provider:

Open communication with your healthcare provider is paramount for ensuring your safety and optimizing the effectiveness of Saxenda. If you have any concerns or questions regarding your treatment, don't hesitate to reach out to your healthcare provider promptly. Whether it's regarding adverse reactions, challenges with adherence, or fluctuations in weight loss progress, your healthcare provider is there to support you every step of the way.

Remember, your healthcare provider is your ally in your weight loss journey, and their guidance and expertise are invaluable resources. By reporting any concerns or changes in your health status to them, you can work together to address issues proactively and tailor your treatment plan to suit your individual needs.

CONCLUSION

"Saxenda Usage Med Guide" serves as a comprehensive resource for individuals embarking on their journey with Saxenda, a powerful tool in the management of obesity. Throughout this guide, we have delved into crucial aspects of Saxenda usage, offering insights and recommendations to ensure safe and effective treatment.

A. Expected timeline for seeing results:

Understanding the timeline for seeing results is paramount in managing expectations and maintaining motivation. While individual responses may vary, it is generally expected that noticeable changes may occur within the first few weeks of starting Saxenda. However, full results often manifest over several months of consistent use, accompanied by healthy lifestyle modifications.

B. Signs of effectiveness and when to reassess treatment:

Recognizing signs of effectiveness is key to gauging the efficacy of Saxenda therapy. Positive indicators may include gradual weight loss, improved metabolic markers, and enhanced feelings of satiety. However, it is essential to reassess treatment if progress stalls or adverse effects arise. Regular consultations with healthcare providers enable timely adjustments to dosage or treatment plans, ensuring optimal outcomes.

C. Monitoring for adverse reactions:

Vigilant monitoring for adverse reactions is imperative to mitigate potential risks associated with Saxenda usage. While side effects are possible, ranging from mild gastrointestinal discomfort to more severe issues, prompt identification and management are crucial. Regular communication with healthcare providers facilitates the monitoring process, enabling timely intervention and support.

D. Reporting concerns to healthcare provider:

Open communication between patients and healthcare providers is paramount in ensuring safe and effective Saxenda therapy. Patients should feel empowered to report any concerns or adverse reactions promptly. Whether it be unexpected symptoms, changes in health status, or questions regarding treatment, proactive engagement facilitates collaborative decision-making and enhances overall treatment outcomes.

"Saxenda Usage Med Guide" empowers individuals with the

knowledge and tools necessary to navigate their Saxenda journey confidently. By understanding the expected timeline for results, recognizing signs of effectiveness, monitoring for adverse reactions, and fostering open communication with healthcare providers, individuals can harness the full potential of Saxenda in their pursuit of improved health and well-being. Through informed guidance and proactive engagement, we pave the way towards a healthier, happier future.

THE END

www.ingramcontent.com/pod-product-compliance
Lightning Source LLC
Chambersburg PA
CBHW050244230526
45470CB00005B/2106